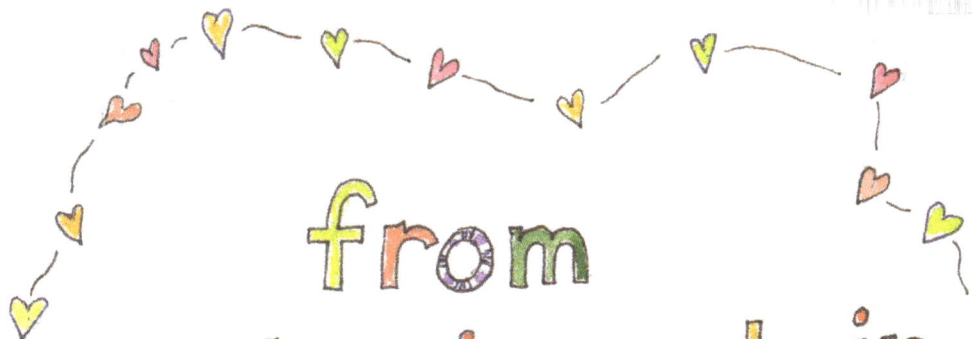

from port wine stain to angel kisses

by Colene Newton
art by Penny Poole Oster

Memoir
BOOKS
Chico, CA

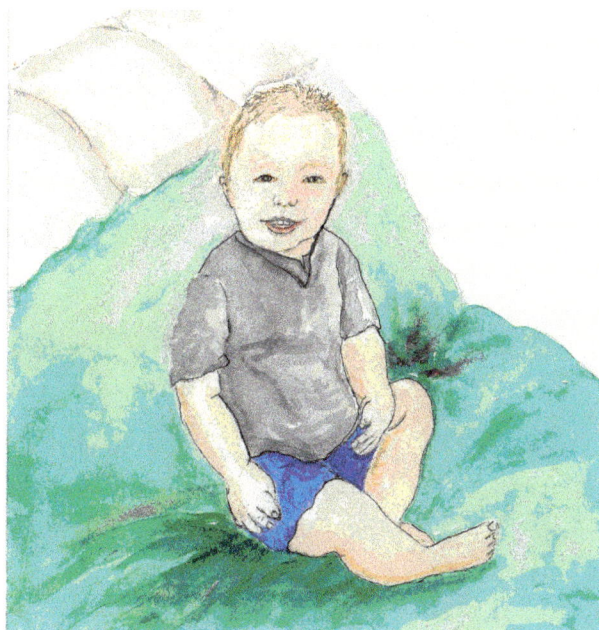

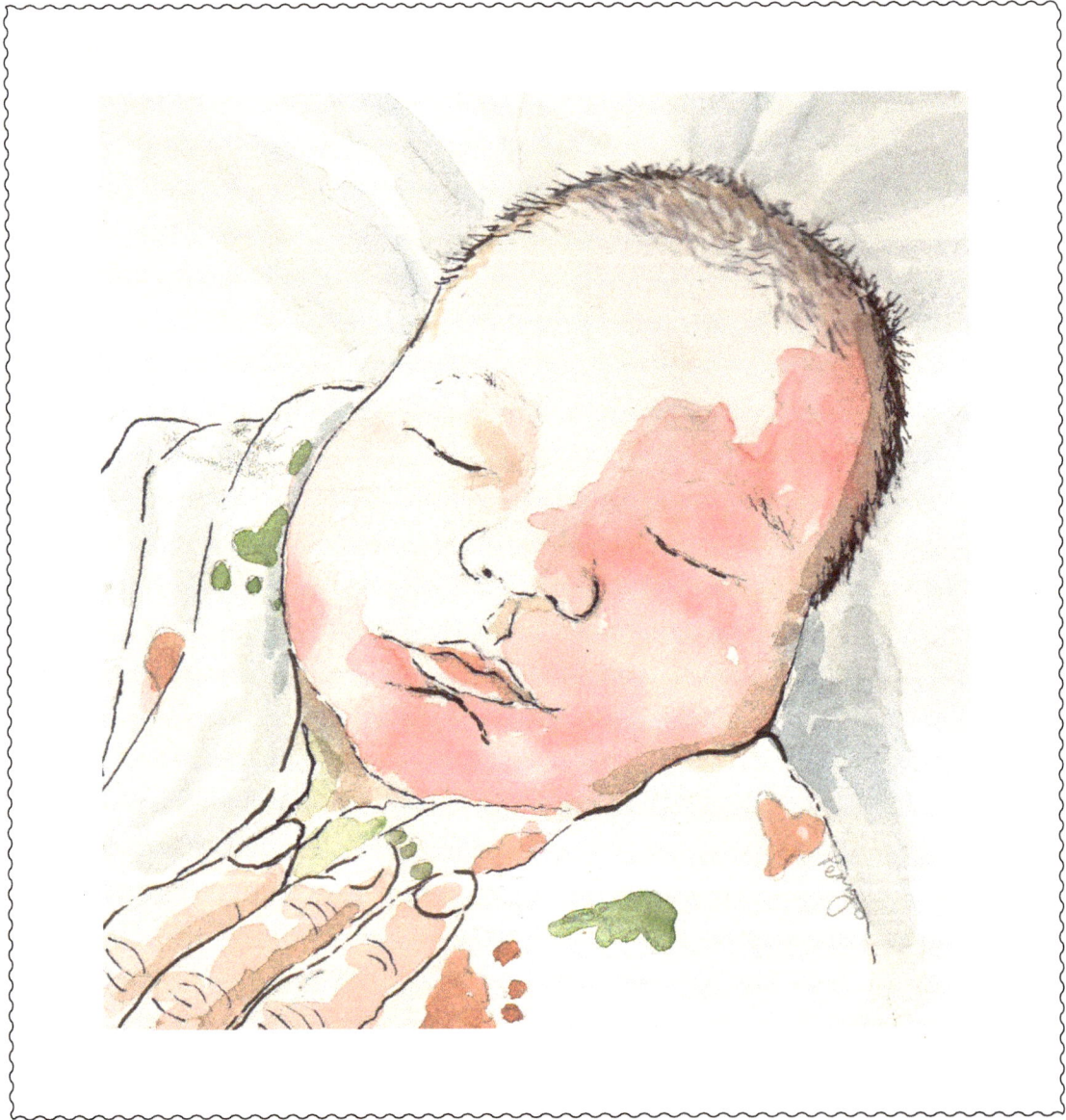

Hello, my name is Leonardo Joshua, but you can call me Leo. I was born with a rare birthmark on my face called *Port Wine Stain*.

Do you have a birthmark anywhere?

My *Port Wine Stain* covers half of my face including one eye and over my brain, which means I also have something called *Sturge-Weber Syndrome.* This makes me even more rare. There are not that many people born with this.

Let me try to explain - have you ever watched a football game? Did you see all those people in the stadium? Well out of all those people only one of them would have *Sturge-Weber Syndrome.* So, I think that makes me really special.

Is there something that makes you special too?

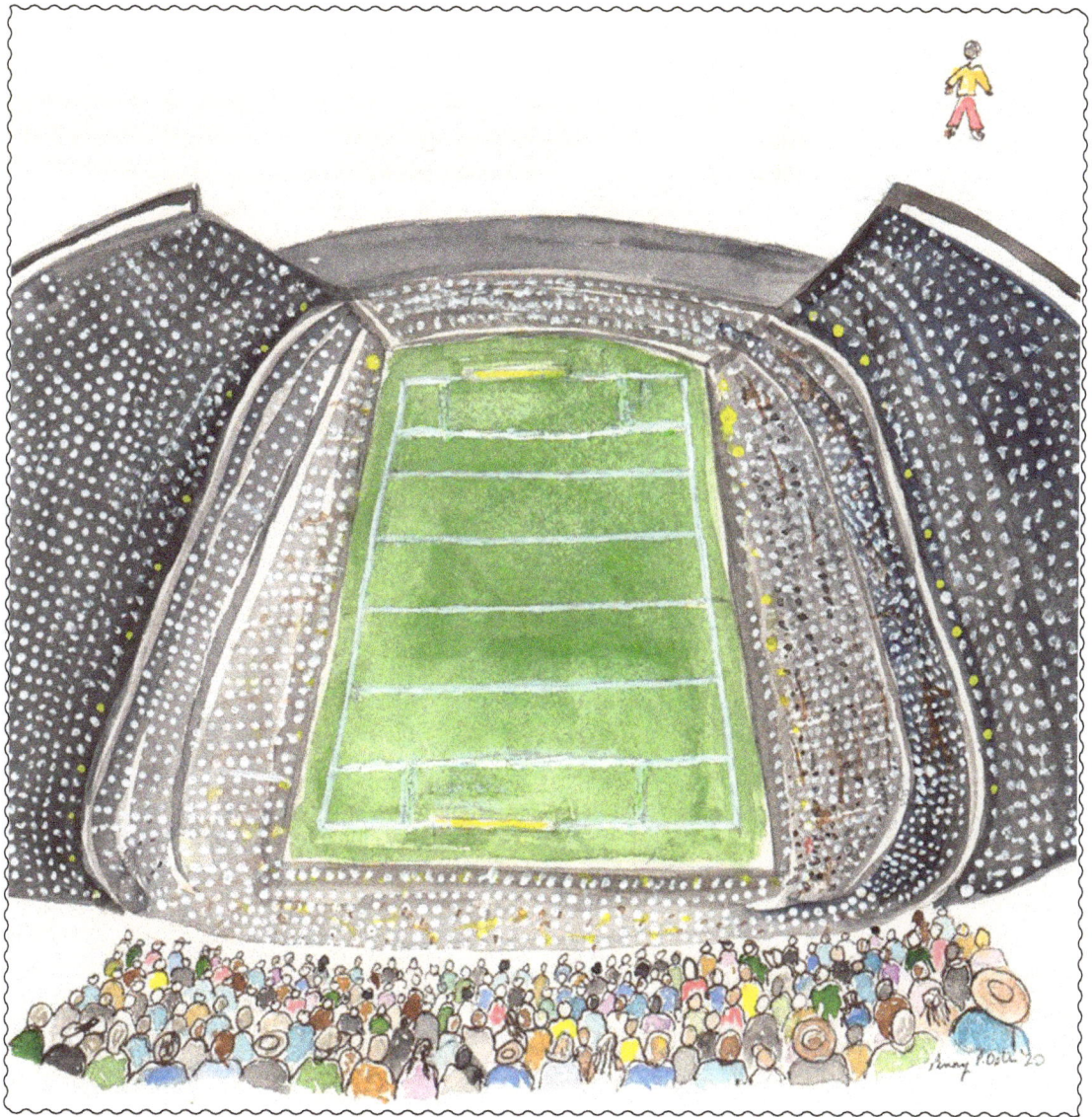

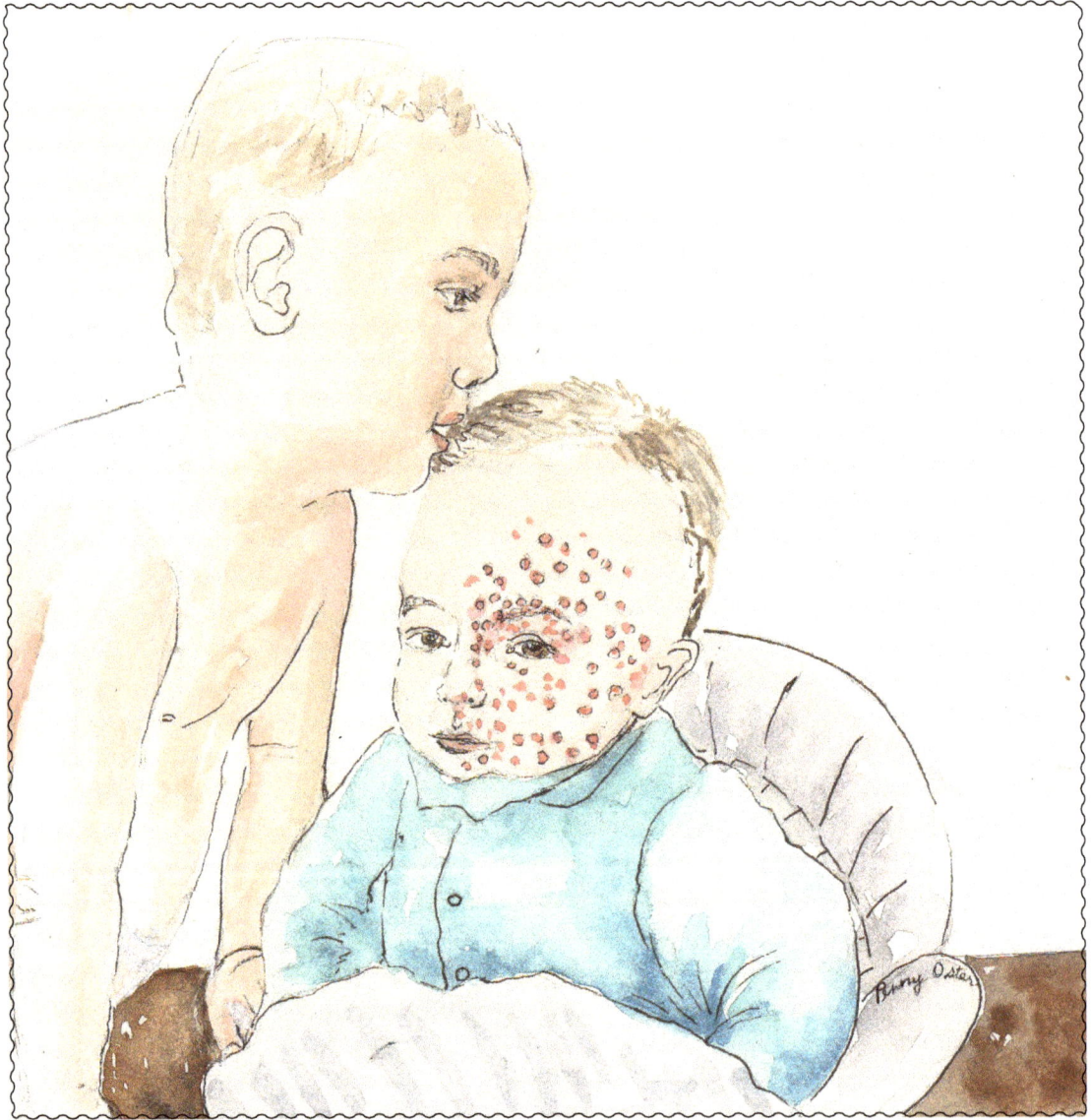

Beny Oster

Sometimes my mom takes me to an office where I get laser treatments on my face to help get rid of the redness. The lasers feel like someone is taking a rubber band and snapping it on my face; it hurts, but only for a second. This is when I have to be really brave. I have had 30 laser treatments!

Afterwards I have polka dots on my face; my mom and my brother call them my Angel Kisses.

Have you ever had to be really brave?

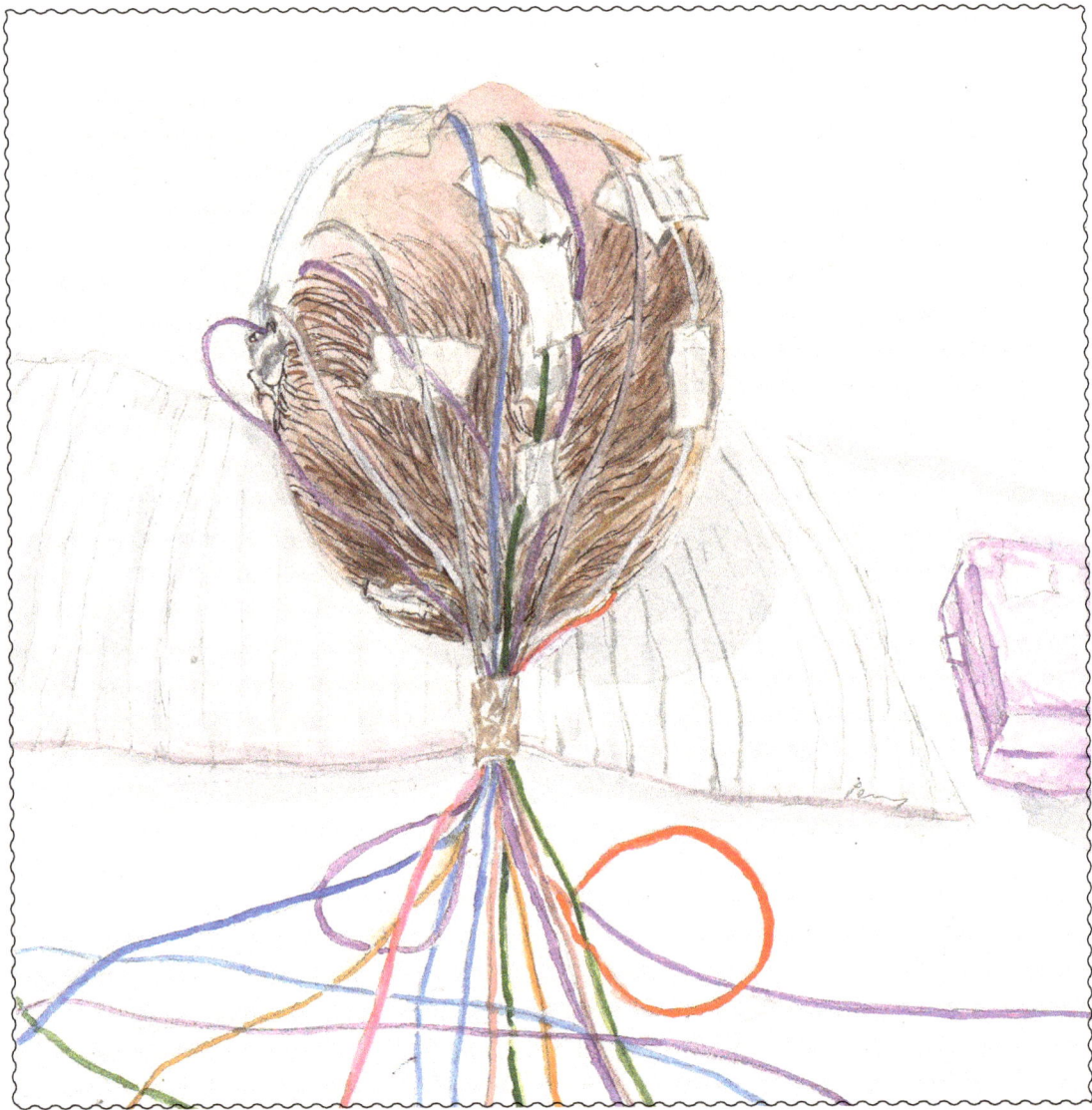

When I was only three months old, I had to go to the hospital to have something called an *EEG* and an *MRI*. I have no idea what they are, but it made my mom cry, a lot. The nurse put colored wires on my head as I slept.

Because of the results I have to take some medicine to keep me from having something called a *seizure*.

I bet some of you have to take medicine too; some medicines taste yucky, but they help us get better.

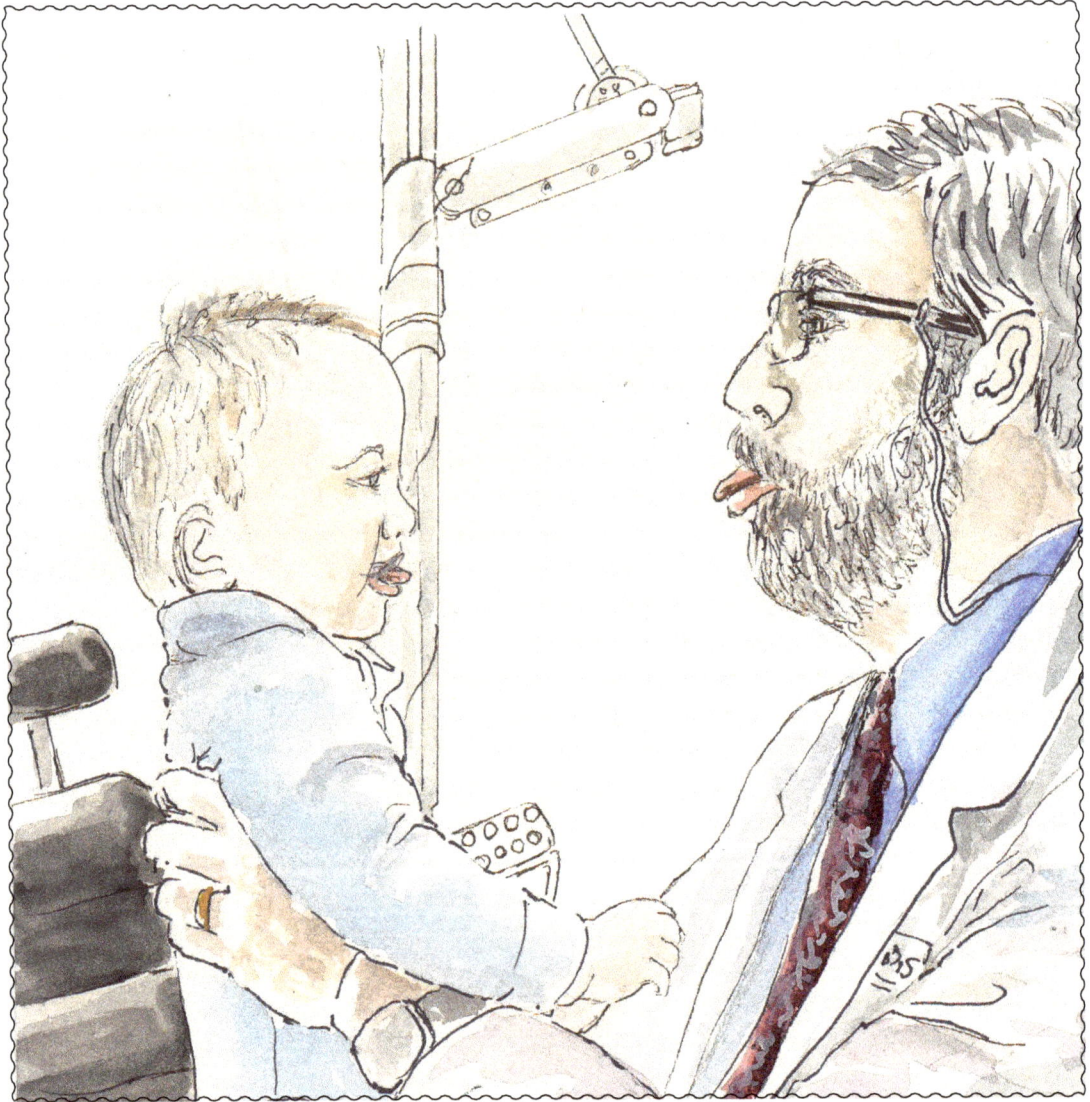

Every three months I visit Dr. Brandt, my eye doctor. He checks my eye pressure for a thing called *glaucoma*. He and I like to make faces at each other, which makes us both giggle.

I bet you visit the doctor sometimes; next time try to make silly faces and see if you giggle too.

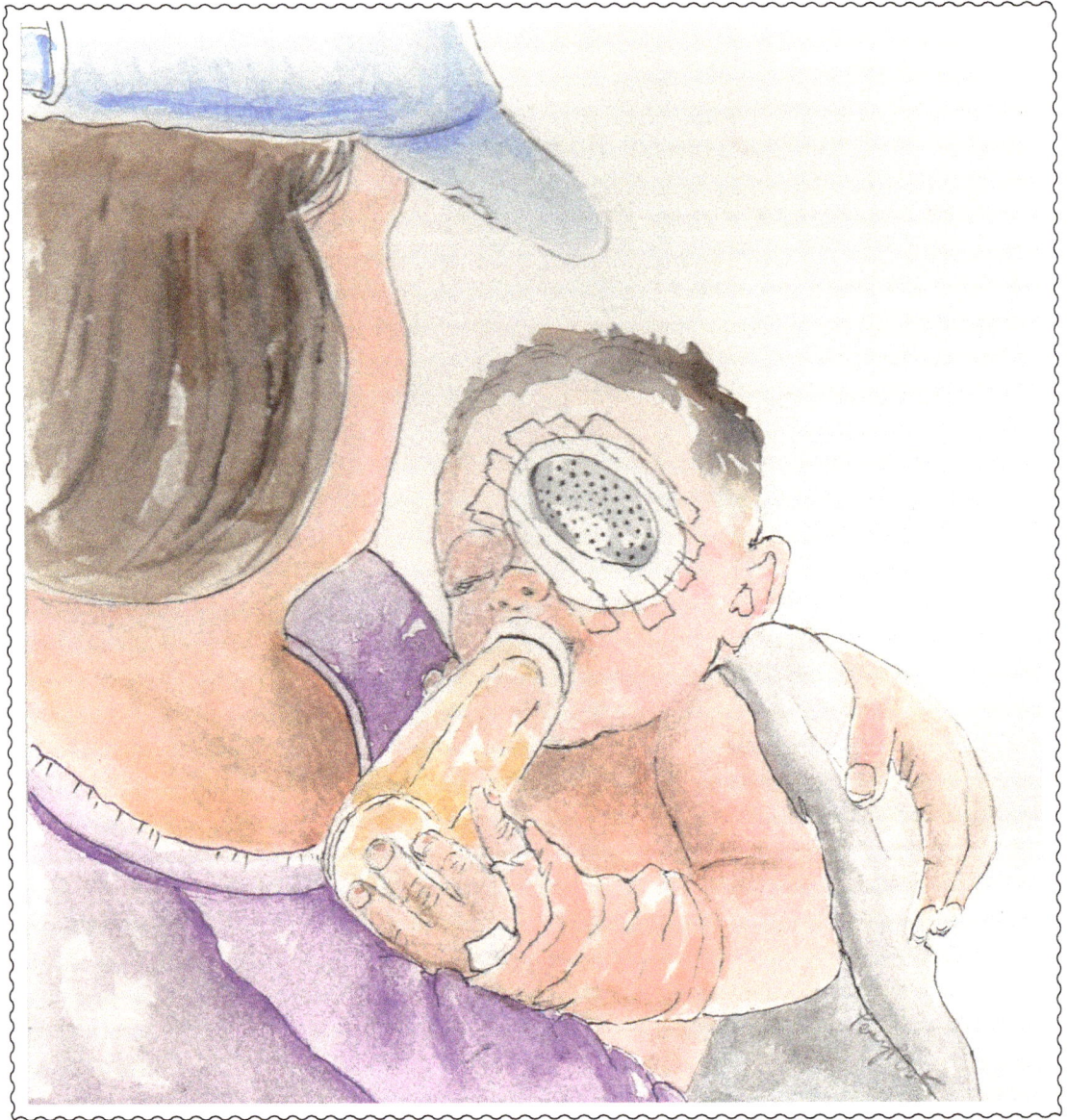

Dr. Brandt put a thing in my eye called a *shunt* to help relieve the pressure. It is like a very, very, very, tiny straw that he carefully placed behind my eye. When I woke up from this surgery, I had an eye patch I got to wear, just like a real pirate.

Do you like to dress up like a pirate?

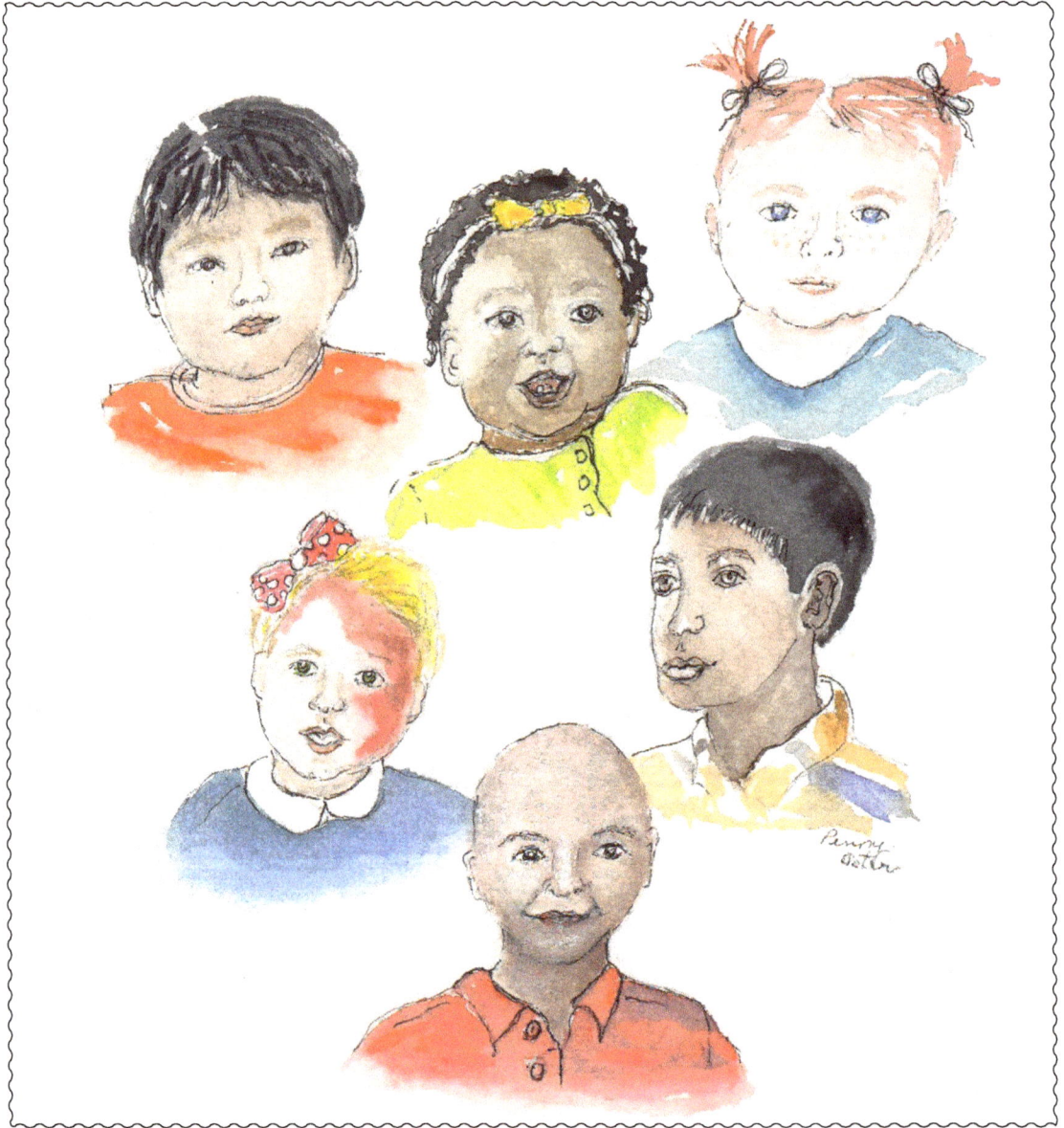

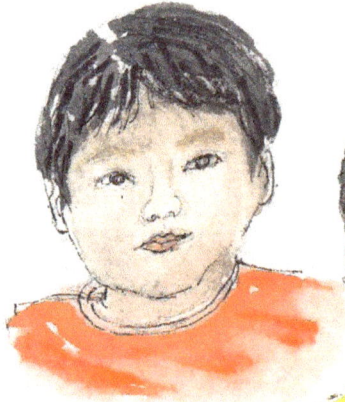

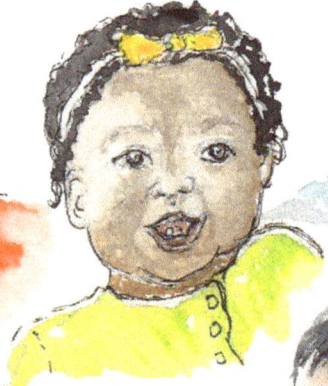

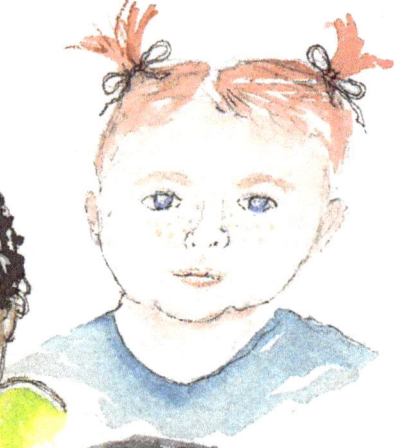

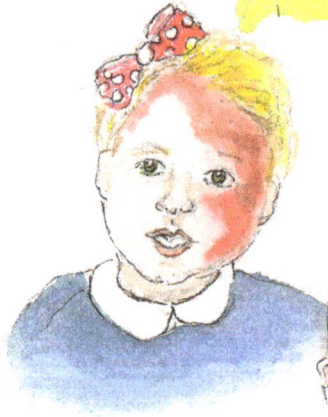

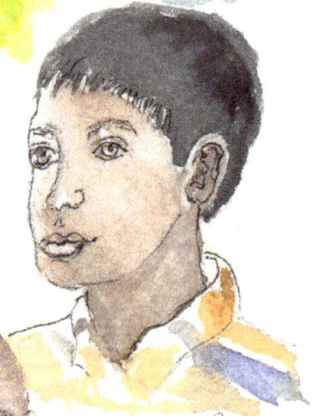

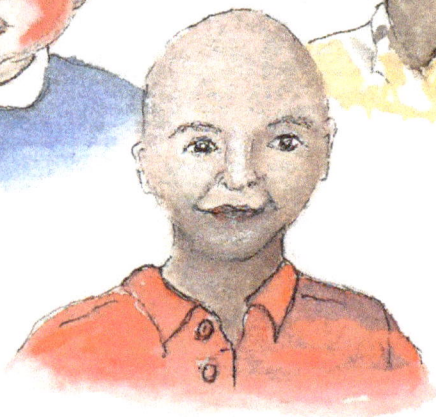

I am unique in so many ways, but so are you. Whether you have curly hair or no hair, a birthmark like me or maybe just a few freckles, we are all different and that's what makes us special. So next time you see someone that is different than you...

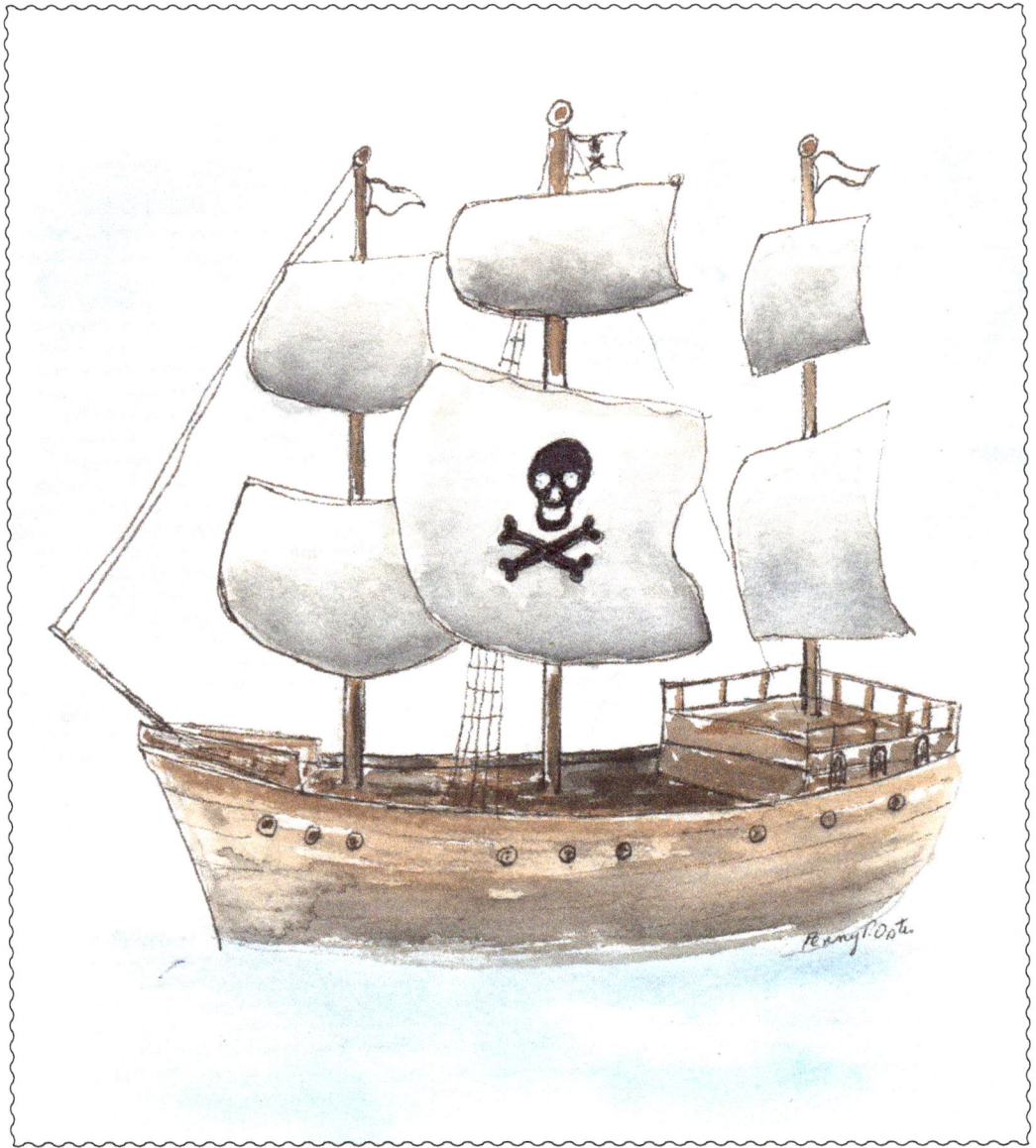

... ask them if they want to play pirates. Chances are, they probably will!

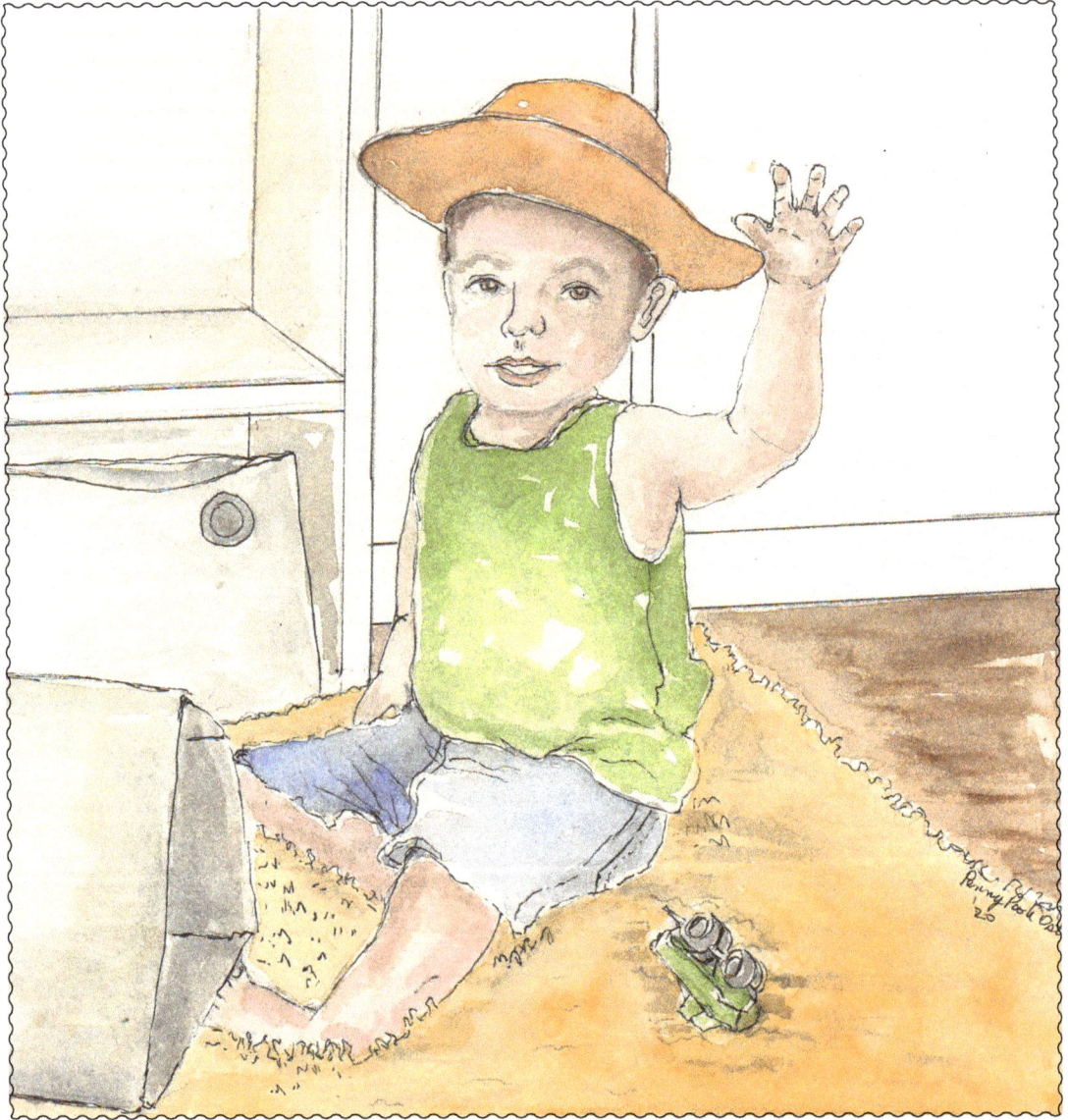

Medical Information

Port Wine Stain A port wine stain (nevus flammeus) is a discoloration of the human skin caused by a vascular anomaly (a capillary malformation in the skin). They are so named for their coloration, which is similar in color to port wine, a fortified red wine from Portugal. A port wine stain is a capillary malformation, seen at birth. Port wine stains always persist throughout life. The area of skin affected grows in proportion to general growth.

Port wine stains occur most often on the face but can appear anywhere on the body, particularly on the neck, upper trunk, arms and legs. Early stains are usually flat and pink in appearance. As the child matures, the color may deepen to a dark red or purplish color. In adulthood, thickening of the lesion or the development of small lumps may occur. Port wine stains may be part of a syndrome such as Sturge–Weber syndrome or Klippel–Trénaunay–Weber syndrome.

Sturge-Weber Syndrome sometimes referred to as encephalotrigeminal angiomatosis, is a rare congenital neurological and skin disorder. It is one of the Phakomatoses and is often associated with port wine stains of the face, glaucoma, seizures, intellectual disability, and ipsilateral leptomeningeal angioma (cerebral malformations and tumors). Sturge–Weber syndrome can be classified into three different types. Type 1 includes facial and leptomeningeal angiomas as well as the possibility of glaucoma or choroidal lesions. Normally, only one side of the brain is affected.

This type is the most common. Type 2 involvement includes a facial angioma (port wine stain) with a possibility of glaucoma developing. There is no evidence of brain involvement. Symptoms can show at any time beyond the initial diagnosis of the facial angioma. The symptoms can include glaucoma, cerebral blood flow abnormalities and headaches. More research is needed on this type of Sturge-Weber syndrome. Type 3 has leptomeningeal angioma involvement exclusively. The facial angioma is absent and glaucoma rarely occurs. This type is only diagnosed via brain scan.

Laser treatments The pulsed dye laser in conjunction with cryogen spray cooling ("dynamic cooling device" or "DCD") is now the treatment of choice for Port Wine Stain. Yellow light produced by the pulsed dye laser penetrates up to 2 mm into the skin and is preferentially absorbed by hemoglobin within the dilated Port Wine Stain blood vessels. The heat within the vessel lumen causes blood vessel damage which is evidenced by intense purpura ("bruised" appearance of the skin). Several treatment sessions spaced at 4-8 week intervals are required for maximum efficacy. The number of treatments required for maximum Port Wine Stain fading can be variable and unpredictable. Treatment side effects are mainly limited to post-operative swelling and purpura, which generally resolves within 2 weeks. With the addition of cryogen spray cooling, the risks of scarring or changes in the normal skin pigmentation are minimal after pulsed dye laser therapy performed by an experienced physician.

MRI Magnetic resonance imaging is a medical imaging technique used in radiology to form pictures of the anatomy and the physiological processes of the body.

EEG An electroencephalogram is a test used to evaluate the electrical activity in the brain. Brain cells communicate with each other through electrical impulses.

Seizure A seizure is a sudden, uncontrolled electrical disturbance in the brain. It can cause changes in your behavior, movements or feelings, and in levels of consciousness.

Glaucoma Glaucoma is a group of eye conditions that damage the optic nerve, the health of which is vital for good vision. This damage is often caused by an abnormally high pressure in your eye.

James Brandt, MD at UC Davis, Sacramento, CA; his clinical practice is limited to the diagnosis and management of all forms of glaucoma, with a particular focus on infantile and pediatric glaucoma.

The Vascular Birthmarks Foundation www.birthmark.org

Hunter Nelson Sturge-Weber Syndrome Center
www.KennedyKrieger.org

Visit **www.ShawntelNewton.com** for more of my real-life story. —Leo

A portion of the sales from this book will go to Sturge-Weber Syndrome research.

www.ingramcontent.com/pod-product-compliance
Lightning Source LLC
Chambersburg PA
CBHW041429270326
41933CB00023B/3492